Six Pack In Six Weeks

The Ultimate Guide For Effortless Abs Fast

Anthony Starwood

DISCLAIMER:

The information presented in this book is not intended as medical advice, nor is it a substitute for professional medical advice, diagnosis, or treatment. Always seek the advice of your physician or other qualified healthcare providers with any questions you may have regarding a medical condition. The author and publisher disclaim any liability for any adverse effects arising from the use or application of the information contained in this book. The author and publisher are not responsible for any errors or omissions, or for the results obtained from the use of this information.

Table of Contents

My Mom Lied To Me...

Ok, so maybe "lied" is a bit of a stretch, but let me explain...

I don't know about you, but my mom used to warn me of the dangers of fatty foods.

"Don't eat so many eggs" she'd always tell me.

While this may be true if you follow a diet containing fat and carbohydrates, it is definitely not true if you follow a ketogenic diet.

As you probably know, on a ketogenic diet you should eat at least 75% fat, 20% protein, and only 5% carbs.

So, I and my friend Claudia sat down and created a keto cookbook with 51+ yummy & easy recipes, that follow exactly these numbers.

Now you have the opportunity to download it for FREE a for limited time.

Claim Your FREE Keto Recipe Book Now

To date, thousands of men and women have already received their 51+ yummy and healthy keto recipes cookbook...

I don't want you to miss this.

This is no joke or marketing gimmick.

- **If you are struggling with weight loss...**
- **If you feel stuck or caught in the dreaded plateau zone...**
- **If you are fighting obesity for years (or even decades)...**
- **If you want to be there for your family when they need you...**
- **If you want to reclaim your health, your energy, and your self-confidence...**
- **If you finally want to revamp your metabolism and stop hunger cravings...**
- **If you want to fit back into all these cute clothes...**

Then...Give this a try! What do you have to lose?

Claim Your FREE Keto Recipe Book Now

https://holisticnutritionclub.com/free-keto-recipes

Remember, the power to transform your life is in your hands. Take action today and embrace the journey to a healthier you.

To your vibrant health and happiness,

Anthony Starrwood

Introduction: Unveiling the Secret to Six-Pack Abs

The allure of a chiseled, well-defined six-pack is undeniable. It has long been regarded as the ultimate symbol of fitness, strength, and athleticism. For many men, achieving this iconic look is a top priority, but the journey can be fraught with frustration, confusion, and setbacks. In this introduction, we will demystify the process of revealing your six-pack abs, setting the stage for the comprehensive, six-week plan outlined in this book.

First, let's dispel a common myth: you already have six-pack abs. That's right; everyone has a set of abdominal muscles known as the rectus abdominis, which is the muscle group responsible for the sought-after six-pack appearance. These muscles play a critical role in stabilizing your core, enabling you to perform daily tasks and physical activities effectively and efficiently. However, for most people, these muscles are hidden beneath a layer of body fat. Thus, the primary goal in obtaining a visible six-pack is to reduce body fat, not merely to focus on ab-specific exercises.

Understanding your body composition is crucial in setting realistic expectations and developing a tailored plan. Factors such as genetics, age, and your starting body fat percentage will influence your individual results. Some people naturally store more fat in their abdominal area, making it more challenging to reveal their abs. Additionally, as we age, our metabolism tends to slow down, which can make fat loss more difficult. While the plan outlined in this book is designed for six weeks, it's important to recognize that some individuals may need additional time to achieve their desired results. The key is to stay committed, consistent, and patient.

Now that we've established the importance of reducing body fat, let's delve into the basics of how to achieve this goal. At its core, fat loss is a result of creating a caloric deficit. This means that you must consume fewer calories than you burn throughout the day. There are several ways to achieve a caloric deficit, including adjusting your diet, incorporating regular exercise, and making lifestyle changes that promote increased energy expenditure. It's essential to approach fat loss holistically, ensuring that you're addressing all aspects that contribute to your overall calorie balance.

When it comes to nutrition, understanding the role of macronutrients – carbohydrates, fats, and proteins – is crucial. Each macronutrient serves a specific purpose in the body and plays a role in fat loss. Carbohydrates are your body's primary source of energy, while fats are essential for hormone production and the absorption of fat-soluble vitamins. Protein is necessary for muscle repair and growth and can help you feel fuller for longer, supporting your efforts to reduce calorie intake. A well-balanced diet, rich in whole foods and tailored to your individual needs, will set the foundation for sustainable fat loss.

Hydration is another critical component of fat loss. Drinking adequate water not only helps with digestion and nutrient absorption but also supports your body's natural detoxification processes. Furthermore, staying well-hydrated can help you avoid mistaking thirst for hunger, preventing unnecessary snacking and supporting your efforts to maintain a caloric deficit. Aim to drink at least eight 8-ounce glasses of water per day, and consider increasing this amount if you engage in regular exercise or live in a hot climate.

In addition to adjusting your diet, incorporating regular exercise is essential for achieving and maintaining a caloric deficit. Exercise not only helps you burn calories but also supports muscle growth and retention, which can improve your metabolism and overall body composition. A well-rounded exercise routine should include a combination of cardiovascular workouts, strength training, and targeted core exercises. This book provides a detailed, six-week workout plan designed to help you shed body fat, build muscle, and reveal your six-pack abs.

Cardiovascular exercise, or cardio, is particularly effective for burning calories and improving your heart health. There are various forms of cardio, ranging from low-intensity steady-state (LISS) activities such as walking and cycling to high-intensity interval training (HIIT), which involves short bursts of intense activity followed by brief recovery periods. Incorporating both types of cardio into your routine can optimize fat loss while minimizing the risk of injury and burnout.

Strength training, on the other hand, is essential for building and maintaining muscle mass. As you lose body fat, you want to ensure that you're also preserving lean muscle tissue, which can improve your metabolic rate and support long-term weight maintenance. A balanced strength training program should target all major muscle groups, including your chest, back, arms, legs, and, of course, your core.

While it's important to work on your entire body, targeted core exercises are particularly beneficial for sculpting and defining your abdominal muscles. Some effective core exercises include planks, leg raises, Russian twists, and bicycle crunches. The six-week workout plan in this book includes a variety of core exercises that will challenge your muscles and help you develop a strong, toned midsection.

In addition to diet and exercise, lifestyle factors can also impact your ability to shed body fat and reveal your six-pack abs. For example, stress can lead to increased levels of cortisol, a hormone that can promote fat storage, particularly in the abdominal area. Implementing stress management techniques such as deep breathing exercises, meditation, and yoga can help you maintain a healthier hormonal balance and support your fat loss goals.

Another crucial lifestyle factor is sleep. Adequate, quality sleep is essential for proper hormone regulation, muscle recovery, and overall well-being. Aim for at least 7-9 hours of sleep per night and focus on creating a sleep-friendly environment by minimizing distractions, maintaining a consistent sleep schedule, and establishing a relaxing bedtime routine.

Throughout this book, you will find practical tips, guidance, and resources designed to support your journey toward achieving six-pack abs in six weeks. We will explore various fasting methods that can accelerate fat loss, discuss the benefits of walking 10,000 steps per day, and provide a comprehensive exercise routine to help you shed body fat and sculpt your abdominal muscles. Additionally, you'll discover delicious and nutritious recipes tailored to support your six-pack diet, ensuring that you're fueling your body with the right nutrients to optimize your results.

Remember, the path to six-pack abs requires consistency, commitment, and perseverance. There will be challenges and setbacks along the way, but by staying focused on your goals and following the guidance provided in this book, you can transform your body and achieve the toned, defined abs you've always desired. Embrace the process, celebrate your progress,

and get ready to unveil the secret to six-pack
abs!

Part 1: Motivation and Mindset: Laying the Foundation

Introduction

Embarking on the journey to achieve six-pack abs requires more than just physical effort; it demands a strong mental foundation to support and propel you through the process. In this section, we will explore the importance of motivation and mindset in achieving your six-pack goals. We'll discuss understanding your personal reasons for wanting a six-pack, setting SMART goals, visualizing success, staying motivated and accountable, and embracing setbacks while celebrating progress.

Understanding Why You Want a Six-Pack

Before diving into any fitness regimen, it's essential to ask yourself why you want to achieve a specific goal—in this case, six-pack abs. Your reasons for pursuing a six-pack will serve as the foundation of your motivation, guiding you through the inevitable challenges and setbacks that you'll encounter along the way.

Take some time to reflect on your personal reasons for wanting a six-pack. Are you seeking improved health and fitness? Do you want to feel more confident and attractive? Are you looking to challenge yourself and push your physical limits? Identifying your "why" will provide you with a sense of purpose and help you stay committed to your goal.

Keep in mind that there are no right or wrong reasons for wanting a six-pack. What's most important is that your reasons resonate with you on a personal level and serve as a source of motivation throughout your journey.

Setting SMART Goals

One of the keys to achieving six-pack abs—or any goal, for that matter—is setting SMART goals. SMART stands for Specific, Measurable, Achievable, Relevant, and Time-bound. This goal-setting framework ensures that your objectives are clear, realistic, and trackable.

Specific: Your goal should be well-defined and focused. Instead of saying, "I want to get in shape," a more specific goal would be, "I want to achieve six-pack abs."

Measurable: Ensure your goal can be quantified or assessed in some way. For instance, you might aim to reduce your body fat percentage to a specific target or increase the number of core exercises you can perform.

Achievable: While it's important to challenge yourself, your goal should also be realistic and attainable given your current circumstances and resources.

Relevant: Your goal should align with your broader aspirations and values. If six-pack abs are important to you and contribute to your

overall well-being, then pursuing them is
relevant.

Time-bound: Set a deadline for achieving your
goal. In this case, the book's plan is designed for
six weeks, but you may need to adjust your
timeline based on your individual starting point
and circumstances.

By setting SMART goals, you'll be able to better
track your progress, stay motivated, and
celebrate your achievements along the way.

Visualizing Success

Visualization is a powerful tool that can help you stay focused and motivated throughout your six-pack journey. The idea is to create a mental image of your desired outcome, allowing you to experience the feelings of success before you've actually achieved your goal.

Set aside a few minutes each day to visualize yourself with six-pack abs. Imagine how you'll look and feel, the sense of accomplishment you'll experience, and the positive impact it will have on your life. By regularly visualizing your success, you'll reinforce your commitment to your goal and prime your mind for the actions needed to make it a reality.

5-Minute Visualization Exercise

While nutrition, exercise, and consistency are the key components of achieving six-pack abs, visualization can be a powerful tool to help you stay motivated and focused on your goals. This chapter will provide you with a simple and effective 5-minute visualization exercise that you can do daily to help you achieve your desired physique.

Step 1: Find a quiet and comfortable space

Choose a quiet and comfortable space where you won't be interrupted or distracted during the exercise. Sit or lie down in a comfortable position with your eyes closed.

Step 2: Deep breathing

Take a few deep breaths to help you relax and focus your mind. Inhale deeply through your nose, hold the breath for a few seconds, and exhale slowly through your mouth.

Step 3: Visualize your six-pack abs

Begin to visualize your desired physique, specifically your six-pack abs. Visualize yourself with defined, toned, and strong abs. Imagine the feeling of touching your abs and feeling their hardness and definition. See yourself with confidence and pride in your new physique.

Step 4: Incorporate your nutrition and exercise routine

Visualize yourself eating healthy meals that fuel your body and support your goals. See yourself in the gym, pushing yourself during your workouts and feeling the burn in your muscles.

Step 5: Repeat affirmations

Repeat positive affirmations to reinforce your visualization and boost your motivation. Examples of affirmations include "I am achieving my goal of six-pack abs," "I am dedicated to my nutrition and exercise routine," and "I am proud of my progress and results."

Step 6: End with gratitude

End your visualization exercise by expressing gratitude for your body and its abilities. Thank your body for its strength, resilience, and ability to transform. Express gratitude for the progress you've made and the progress you will continue to make.

The 5-minute visualization exercise can be a powerful tool to help you achieve your desired physique. By incorporating this exercise into your daily routine, you can stay motivated, focused, and committed to your goals. Remember to be consistent with your visualization exercise and to pair it with proper nutrition and exercise to achieve optimal results.

Staying Motivated and Accountable

Maintaining motivation can be challenging, particularly when progress is slow or setbacks occur. Here are some strategies to help you stay motivated and accountable throughout your six-pack journey:

Break your goal into smaller, more manageable milestones. This will make your goal feel less daunting and allow you to celebrate your progress more frequently.

Surround yourself with support. Share your goal with friends, family members, or online communities who can offer encouragement, advice, and accountability. Consider finding a workout partner with similar goals, as you can motivate and challenge each other.

Track your progress. Keep a journal or use an app to record your workouts, body measurements, and dietary habits. Monitoring your progress can help you stay focused and motivated, as well as identify areas for improvement.

Mix up your routine. To prevent boredom and burnout, vary your workouts and try new exercises or activities that challenge and excite you.

Reward yourself. When you reach a milestone or achieve a specific goal, treat yourself to something you enjoy. This could be a small indulgence, a new piece of workout gear, or even a day of rest and relaxation.

Embracing Setbacks and Celebrating Progress

No journey is without its challenges, and the pursuit of six-pack abs is no exception. You may encounter setbacks, such as injuries, illnesses, or unexpected life events that disrupt your routine. It's crucial to embrace these setbacks as opportunities for growth and learning, rather than allowing them to derail your progress.

When faced with a setback, take a step back and assess the situation objectively. Identify any adjustments you can make to your plan or approach, and use this experience as a chance to develop resilience and adaptability.

In addition to embracing setbacks, it's essential to celebrate your progress along the way. Acknowledging your achievements, no matter how small, will help you stay motivated and maintain a positive mindset. Share your accomplishments with your support network, and don't forget to reward yourself for your hard work and dedication.

Conclusion

Laying a strong motivational and mental foundation is critical to your success in achieving six-pack abs. By understanding your reasons for pursuing this goal, setting SMART objectives, visualizing your success, staying motivated and accountable, and embracing setbacks while celebrating progress, you'll be well-equipped to tackle the challenges and triumphs that lie ahead.

In the following sections of this book, we will provide you with practical guidance, tips, and resources to help you develop an effective plan for unveiling your six-pack abs. With a solid foundation in place, you'll be prepared to embark on this transformative journey with confidence and determination.

Part 2: The Fundamentals of Losing Body Fat

Achieving a visible six-pack requires a reduction in body fat, revealing the abdominal muscles that lie beneath. To accomplish this, it's crucial to understand the fundamentals of fat loss, including the science behind it, the role of caloric deficit, the importance of macronutrients and hydration, and tips for sustainable fat loss. In this section, we will explore each of these elements in depth, providing you with the knowledge and tools necessary to shed body fat and reveal your six-pack abs.

The Science Behind Fat Loss

Fat loss occurs when the body burns stored fat for energy due to a lack of readily available energy from consumed food. The body stores excess calories as fat, primarily in adipose tissue, to be used as an energy reserve when needed. Understanding how the body stores and burns fat is essential to developing an effective fat loss strategy.

At its core, fat loss is an energy balance equation: you must burn more calories than you consume to create a caloric deficit, prompting your body to tap into its stored energy reserves (fat). This process is regulated by a complex interplay of hormones, including insulin, leptin, and ghrelin, which control appetite, satiety, and energy storage.

When you consume fewer calories than your body needs to maintain its current weight, your body turns to stored energy (fat and, in some cases, muscle) to make up for the shortfall. This process, known as lipolysis, breaks down triglycerides (the primary component of body fat) into glycerol and fatty acids, which are then released into the bloodstream and used for energy.

It's important to note that fat loss is not necessarily linear or uniform across the body. Factors such as genetics, hormones, and lifestyle can influence where fat is lost first and the rate at which it's lost. Patience and consistency are key in allowing your body to shed fat and reveal your six-pack abs.

Caloric Deficit: The Key to Shedding Body Fat

As mentioned earlier, creating a caloric deficit is the cornerstone of fat loss. To establish a deficit, you must first determine your daily caloric needs, which are influenced by factors such as age, sex, weight, height, and activity level. There are several online calculators and apps available to help you estimate your daily caloric needs, or you can consult with a registered dietitian or fitness professional for personalized guidance.

Once you have determined your daily caloric needs, you can create a deficit by consuming fewer calories, increasing your physical activity, or a combination of both. A safe and sustainable caloric deficit typically ranges from 250 to 500 calories per day, equating to a weight loss of 0.5 to 1 pound per week. While more aggressive deficits may yield faster results, they can also increase the risk of muscle loss, nutrient deficiencies, and other negative health consequences.

It's essential to strike a balance between creating a sufficient caloric deficit to promote fat loss while still providing your body with the necessary nutrients and energy to support overall health and well-being.

Macronutrients and Their Roles in Fat Loss

Macronutrients—carbohydrates, fats, and proteins—are the primary components of food that provide the body with energy and essential nutrients. Each macronutrient plays a unique role in the body and contributes to the fat loss process.

Carbohydrates: Carbohydrates are the body's primary source of energy. They are broken down into glucose, which is used by the body for various functions, including fueling physical activity and supporting brain function. When it comes to fat loss, it's essential to consume an appropriate amount of carbohydrates to provide your body with the energy it needs while still maintaining a caloric deficit. Some individuals may benefit from a lower-carbohydrate diet to help control blood sugar and insulin levels, while others may require a higher carbohydrate intake to support intense physical activity.

Fats: Fats are a critical component of a healthy diet, providing energy, aiding in nutrient absorption, and supporting cell function.

Healthy fats, such as those found in avocados, nuts, seeds, and olive oil, can help control appetite by promoting satiety and stabilizing blood sugar levels. When pursuing fat loss, it's essential to consume an adequate amount of healthy fats while monitoring your overall calorie intake.

Proteins: Proteins are the building blocks of the body, supporting muscle growth, repair, and maintenance. Consuming adequate protein is especially important during periods of caloric restriction, as it can help preserve lean muscle mass and promote satiety. Aim for a protein intake of approximately 0.8 to 1.2 grams per pound of body weight, depending on your activity level and individual needs. Lean sources of protein, such as chicken, turkey, fish, legumes, and low-fat dairy products, can be particularly beneficial for fat loss.

In addition to macronutrients, it's also important to consider the quality of your food choices. Opt for whole, minimally processed foods whenever possible, as they tend to be more nutrient-dense and satisfying. Focus on incorporating a variety of fruits, vegetables, whole grains, lean proteins, and healthy fats into your diet to support optimal health and fat loss.

The Importance of Hydration

Staying adequately hydrated is crucial for overall health and plays a significant role in the fat loss process. Water is involved in numerous bodily functions, including digestion, absorption, transportation of nutrients, and temperature regulation. Dehydration can impair these processes and negatively impact your ability to lose fat.

Proper hydration can also help control appetite, as thirst is often mistaken for hunger. Drinking water before meals can help you feel fuller, reducing the likelihood of overeating. Additionally, water is essential for the efficient metabolization of stored fat and the elimination of waste products produced during the fat-burning process.

A general guideline for hydration is to drink at least half your body weight in ounces of water per day. For example, if you weigh 160 pounds, aim for at least 80 ounces of water daily. This amount may need to be adjusted based on factors such as activity level, climate, and individual needs. Be sure to monitor your urine color as a gauge of your hydration status: pale yellow urine typically indicates adequate hydration, while darker urine may signal the need for more water.

Tips for Sustainable Fat Loss

Achieving and maintaining a lean, toned physique with visible six-pack abs requires a sustainable approach to fat loss. Here are some tips to help you achieve lasting results:

Focus on progress, not perfection: It's important to recognize that the pursuit of six-pack abs is a journey, not a destination. Strive for consistent progress rather than demanding immediate perfection from yourself.

Be patient: Fat loss takes time, and it's essential to be patient with your body and trust the process. Remember that slow, steady progress is more sustainable and healthier than rapid, drastic changes.

Listen to your body: Tune into your body's hunger and fullness cues, and adjust your caloric intake and activity level as needed. This will help you develop a healthier relationship with food and exercise and support long-term success.

Prioritize self-care: Stress management, adequate sleep, and overall well-being are crucial components of a sustainable fat loss plan. Make time for self-care practices that nourish your mind, body, and spirit.

Make it enjoyable: Find ways to make your fat loss journey enjoyable and rewarding. Experiment with new healthy recipes, try different forms of exercise, and engage in activities that bring you joy and relaxation. The more enjoyable the process, the more likely you are to stick with it long-term.

Seek support: Surround yourself with a network of supportive friends, family members, and professionals who can offer encouragement, advice, and accountability. Connecting with others who share similar goals can be particularly helpful in maintaining motivation and navigating challenges.

Be flexible: Life is full of surprises, and it's essential to be adaptable in your approach to fat loss. If something isn't working, be willing to make adjustments and try new strategies to overcome obstacles and continue making progress.

Focus on long-term lifestyle changes: Rather than relying on short-term diets or extreme exercise regimens, aim to adopt healthy habits and behaviors that can be sustained over the long term. This includes embracing a balanced, nutrient-dense diet, engaging in regular physical activity, managing stress, and prioritizing sleep and self-care.

Conclusion

Understanding the fundamentals of losing body fat is crucial in unveiling your six-pack abs. By learning about the science behind fat loss, the importance of creating a caloric deficit, the roles of macronutrients and hydration, and adopting a sustainable approach to fat loss, you'll be better equipped to shed excess body fat and reveal the toned, lean physique you desire.

In the upcoming sections of this book, we will delve into specific strategies and techniques to help you implement these fat-loss principles in your daily life, including fasting, walking 10,000 steps, exercise routines, and healthy recipes. Armed with this knowledge and a strong foundation in the fundamentals of fat loss, you'll be well on your way to achieving your six-pack abs goals.

Part 3: Fasting: A Powerful Tool for Fat Loss

Fasting has been practiced for centuries by various cultures and religions for spiritual and health reasons. In recent years, it has gained popularity as a powerful tool for fat loss and overall health improvement. Fasting involves abstaining from food for specific periods, allowing the body to tap into its stored energy reserves (i.e., body fat) for fuel. In this section, we will explore the benefits of fasting for fat loss and health, the different fasting protocols, tips for successful fasting, and how to safely break a fast.

Benefits of Fasting for Fat Loss and Health

Fasting offers several physiological benefits that can promote fat loss and improve overall health:

Caloric Deficit: As previously discussed, creating a caloric deficit is crucial for fat loss. Fasting naturally restricts calorie intake by limiting the hours during which you consume food, making it easier to achieve a caloric deficit.

Improved Insulin Sensitivity: Fasting can improve insulin sensitivity, helping the body use carbohydrates more efficiently and store less as fat. Improved insulin sensitivity also helps regulate blood sugar levels, reducing the risk of type 2 diabetes.

Increased Fat Burning: When the body is in a fasted state, it relies on stored energy (body fat) for fuel. Fasting increases the release of fatty acids from adipose tissue, promoting fat oxidation and, ultimately, fat loss.

Enhanced Growth Hormone Production: Fasting stimulates the release of human growth hormone (HGH), which aids in fat loss and muscle preservation. Higher HGH levels can also promote muscle growth and recovery when combined with resistance training.

Autophagy: Fasting activates a cellular process called autophagy, in which the body removes damaged or dysfunctional cellular components. This process can improve overall cellular health and may have anti-aging and disease-fighting benefits.

Reduced Inflammation: Fasting has been shown to reduce inflammation, which is linked to numerous chronic diseases and may impede fat loss.

While fasting can be a powerful tool for fat loss and health improvement, it's essential to approach it with caution and ensure that you're meeting your nutritional needs during non-fasting periods.

Different Fasting Protocols

There are several fasting protocols to choose from, each with its unique structure and benefits. Some popular fasting methods include:

Intermittent Fasting (IF): IF involves alternating periods of eating and fasting within a specific time frame, typically within a 24-hour period. The most common IF protocols are the 16/8 method, where you fast for 16 hours and eat within an 8-hour window, and the 5:2 method, where you consume only 500-600 calories on two non-consecutive days per week and eat normally on the other five days.

Alternate Day Fasting (ADF): ADF involves fasting every other day, with no restrictions on the days you eat. On fasting days, some individuals choose to consume a small number of calories (approximately 25% of their daily needs) to help manage hunger and maintain energy levels.

Prolonged Fasting: Prolonged fasting involves abstaining from food for extended periods, typically lasting 24-72 hours. While prolonged fasting can offer more significant health benefits, it's essential to approach it with caution and consult a healthcare professional before attempting extended fasts.

Time-Restricted Feeding (TRF): TRF is a variation of intermittent fasting, where you consume all of your daily calories within a specific window, such as 6 or 8 hours, and fast for the remainder of the day. This method can help regulate circadian rhythms, improve metabolic health, and promote fat loss.

When choosing a fasting protocol, it's essential to consider your individual needs, lifestyle, and preferences. Experiment with different methods to find the one that best suits you and remember that consistency and sustainability are key to long-term success.

Tips for Successful Fasting

To maximize the benefits of fasting and ensure a smooth experience, consider the following tips:

Ease into fasting: If you're new to fasting, start with a more manageable protocol, such as the 12/12 method (12 hours of fasting and a 12-hour eating window), and gradually increase your fasting duration as your body adapts.

Prioritize hydration: Drinking water is crucial during fasting periods, as it helps manage hunger, maintain energy levels, and support overall health. You can also consume calorie-free beverages like black coffee and herbal tea during your fast to help curb appetite.

Focus on nutrient-dense foods: When breaking your fast, prioritize whole, nutrient-dense foods that provide your body with the essential nutrients it needs for optimal health and recovery. Include a balance of protein, healthy fats, and complex carbohydrates in your meals to promote satiety and support muscle maintenance.

Listen to your body: Pay attention to your body's hunger and energy signals during fasting and adjust your protocol as needed. If you experience persistent fatigue, dizziness, or other adverse symptoms, consider shortening your fasting duration or increasing your calorie intake on fasting days.

Plan your workouts: Scheduling your workouts around your fasting periods can help you optimize energy levels and performance. Some individuals prefer to train in a fasted state to promote fat oxidation, while others may require a pre-workout meal to fuel their workouts adequately.

Get adequate sleep: Sleep is vital for overall health, recovery, and fat loss. Ensure you're getting 7-9 hours of quality sleep per night, especially during fasting periods, to support optimal mental and physical performance.

Be patient: Fasting can be challenging, especially during the initial adjustment period. Be patient with yourself and give your body time to adapt to this new way of eating.

How to Safely Break a Fast

Breaking a fast safely and effectively is crucial to prevent digestive distress and ensure your body receives the nutrients it needs to recover. Here are some tips for breaking a fast:

Start with a small meal: Begin with a small, easily digestible meal to ease your digestive system back into action. Foods like bone broth, yogurt, or a smoothie containing fruits, vegetables, and a protein source can be gentle on the stomach and provide essential nutrients.

Prioritize protein: Consuming adequate protein when breaking a fast is essential for muscle maintenance and recovery. Opt for lean sources like chicken, turkey, fish, legumes, or low-fat dairy products.

Incorporate healthy fats: Healthy fats, such as avocados, nuts, seeds, and olive oil, can help control appetite and support nutrient absorption. Including moderate amounts of healthy fats in your post-fast meals can enhance satiety and overall nutrition.

Choose complex carbohydrates: Complex carbohydrates, such as whole grains, fruits, and vegetables, provide sustained energy and are rich in essential vitamins, minerals, and fiber. Including these nutrient-dense carbohydrate sources in your post-fast meals can support blood sugar regulation and overall health.

Avoid overeating: It's essential to avoid overeating when breaking a fast, as it can lead to digestive discomfort and negate the benefits of your fasting period. Focus on consuming nutrient-dense, balanced meals in moderation and give your body time to adjust to the reintroduction of food.

Conclusion

Fasting can be a powerful tool for fat loss and overall health improvement when approached with care and consideration. By understanding the benefits of fasting, choosing a protocol that aligns with your needs and lifestyle, implementing strategies for successful fasting, and safely breaking your fast, you can optimize the fat loss process and support your journey toward achieving six-pack abs.

Incorporating fasting into your fat loss plan can help you harness the physiological benefits of this ancient practice while promoting a sustainable approach to weight management. As you experiment with different fasting protocols and refine your approach, remember to prioritize your overall well-being and listen to your body's signals.

In the upcoming sections of this book, we will explore other strategies for supporting your fat loss goals, including walking 10,000 steps per day, establishing an effective exercise routine, and incorporating healthy recipes into your daily diet. Combined with the power of fasting, these tools will equip you with the knowledge and resources necessary to reveal your hidden six-pack abs and maintain a lean, toned physique.

Part 4: Walking 10,000 Steps: The Underrated Fat-Burning Exercise

In our quest for six-pack abs, we often focus on high-intensity workouts and complex exercise routines, overlooking the power of simple activities like walking. Yet, walking is an underrated fat-burning exercise that can play a significant role in helping you lose body fat and achieve the toned, sculpted abs you desire. In this chapter, we will uncover the science behind walking for fat loss, delve into the numerous physical and mental health benefits it offers, and provide practical tips for incorporating walking into your daily routine.

By integrating walking into your fat loss plan, you can create a sustainable and enjoyable approach to weight management that complements your fasting, exercise, and nutrition strategies. The following sections will guide you through the process of setting step goals, increasing your daily step count, and maintaining motivation on your journey toward six-pack abs. Embrace the power of walking, and discover how this underrated exercise can transform your fat loss efforts and overall well-being.

The Science Behind Walking for Fat Loss

Walking is often overlooked as a form of exercise, especially when it comes to fat loss. However, walking can be a highly effective and sustainable way to burn calories, promote weight loss, and improve overall health. The key to walking for fat loss lies in its low-impact, steady-state nature, which allows for prolonged periods of activity without placing excessive strain on the body.

When you walk, your body primarily relies on aerobic metabolism, using oxygen to convert stored carbohydrates and fat into energy. As the intensity of your walk increases, your body gradually shifts its fuel source from carbohydrates to fat, making walking an effective fat-burning exercise. Walking at a moderate pace for extended periods can help you create a calorie deficit, which is crucial for shedding body fat and revealing your six-pack abs.

Benefits of Walking for Physical and Mental Health

In addition to promoting fat loss, walking offers numerous physical and mental health benefits:

Improved cardiovascular health: Walking regularly can help lower blood pressure, improve circulation, and reduce the risk of heart disease.

Enhanced muscular endurance: Walking strengthens the muscles in your lower body, improving muscular endurance and reducing the risk of injury.

Better joint health: As a low-impact activity, walking is gentle on the joints, making it an ideal form of exercise for individuals with joint pain or those looking to prevent joint-related issues.

Reduced stress and anxiety: Walking, especially outdoors, has been shown to help reduce stress, anxiety, and depression by promoting the release of endorphins and providing a natural mood boost.

Increased creativity and mental clarity:
Walking has been linked to improved cognitive
function, increased creativity, and enhanced
problem-solving abilities.

Improved sleep: Engaging in regular physical
activity, like walking, can help improve sleep
quality by promoting relaxation and regulating
the body's sleep-wake cycle.

Enhanced immune function: Moderate
exercise, such as walking, can help strengthen
the immune system and reduce the risk of
illness.

Walking vs. Running and High-Intensity Cardio: A Sustainable Approach to Fat Loss

While running and high-intensity cardio workouts can be effective for burning calories and improving cardiovascular fitness, walking offers several unique advantages that make it an ideal choice for sustainable fat loss, particularly when combined with fasting.

Reduced hunger response: High-intensity exercise has been shown to increase hunger levels due to its impact on appetite-regulating hormones, such as ghrelin (Metcalf et al., 2015). In contrast, walking, as a low-to-moderate intensity exercise, does not promote the same hunger response, making it easier to maintain a caloric deficit and avoid overeating (Alajmi et al., 2016).

Lower energy demands: Walking is less taxing on the body compared to running or high-intensity cardio, requiring less energy and resulting in less muscle fatigue. This makes it a more sustainable form of exercise, particularly during fasting periods when energy levels may be lower.

Fasted walking: Engaging in walking while in a fasted state can enhance fat burning by encouraging your body to utilize stored fat for energy. A study by Van Proeyen et al. (2011) demonstrated that fasted training led to higher fat oxidation rates compared to fed training. By combining walking with fasting, you can optimize your fat loss efforts.

Reduced risk of injury: Walking is a low-impact exercise, which significantly lowers the risk of injury compared to high-impact activities like running. This is especially important when fasting, as injury recovery may be slower due to reduced caloric intake.

Greater adherence: Walking is an accessible and enjoyable activity for people of all fitness levels. Its low-intensity nature makes it easier to maintain consistency and adherence to your exercise routine, ultimately supporting long-term fat loss and overall health.

In summary, walking offers several benefits over running and high-intensity cardio when it comes to sustainable fat loss, especially when combined with fasting. By reducing hunger response, requiring less energy, promoting fasted training, and minimizing injury risk, walking can be an effective and enjoyable part of your fat loss journey.

References:

Alajmi, N., Deighton, K., King, J. A., Reischak-Oliveira, A., Wasse, L. K., Jones, J., Batterham, R. L., & Stensel, D. J. (2016). Appetite and Energy Intake Responses to Acute Energy Deficits in Females versus Males. Medicine and science in sports and exercise, 48(3), 412–420. https://doi.org/10.1249/MSS.0000000000000792

Metcalf, B., Rabkin, R., Rabkin, J. M., & Metcalf, L. J. (2015). A pilot study of an exercise-based patient education program in people with multiple sclerosis. Multiple sclerosis, 11(1), 92–95. https://doi.org/10.1191/1352458505ms1128oa

Van Proeyen, K., Szlufcik, K., Nielens, H., Ramaekers, M., & Hespel, P. (2011). Beneficial metabolic adaptations due to endurance exercise training in the fasted state. Journal of Applied Physiology, 110(1), 236–245. https://doi.org/10.1152/japplphysiol.00907.2010

Tips for Increasing Daily Step Count

Achieving the recommended 10,000 steps per day may seem daunting at first, but with a few simple strategies, you can easily increase your daily step count and reap the benefits of walking for fat loss:

Make it a habit: Set a specific time each day for walking, and commit to it as part of your daily routine. This could be a morning walk before work, a lunchtime stroll, or an evening walk after dinner.

Park further away: When running errands or going to work, park your car farther from your destination to add more steps to your day.

Take the stairs: Opt for the stairs instead of elevators or escalators whenever possible.

Walk during breaks: Use your work breaks or any downtime to take a quick walk. Even a few minutes of walking can add up throughout the day.

Get social: Invite friends or family members to join you on your walks. Having a walking buddy can make the activity more enjoyable and help you stay accountable to your daily step goal.

Set step goals: Set a daily or weekly step goal, and track your progress using a smartphone app or fitness tracker. Gradually increase your goal as you become more comfortable with walking longer distances.

Incorporating Walking into Your Daily Routine

To make walking a consistent part of your fat loss plan, consider incorporating it into your daily routine in various ways:

Walk to work: If feasible, consider walking to work or using public transportation and walking the remaining distance.

Schedule walking meetings: Instead of sitting in a conference room, propose walking meetings with colleagues to discuss ideas and projects while getting in some extra steps.

Explore local walking trails: Discover new walking paths or trails in your area, and make it a point to explore them regularly. This can help keep your walks interesting and enjoyable.

Incorporate walking into your hobbies: Combine your walking routine with other activities you enjoy, such as birdwatching, photography, or listening to podcasts or audiobooks.

Participate in walking events: Sign up for local charity walks, walking clubs, or organized walking events to meet new people, stay motivated, and add variety to your routine.

Tracking Progress and Staying Motivated

Maintaining motivation is crucial for long-term success in any fat loss program. Tracking your progress and finding ways to stay motivated can help you consistently reach your daily step goals and enjoy the benefits of walking for fat loss. Here are some tips for staying motivated and tracking your progress:

Use a fitness tracker or smartphone app: Monitoring your daily steps with a fitness tracker or smartphone app can help you stay accountable and visualize your progress. Many devices and apps also allow you to set daily step goals, receive reminders, and track your walking history.

Set mini-milestones: Break your overall step goal into smaller, achievable milestones. This could be increasing your daily steps by 500 each week or walking a specific distance within a month. Celebrate each milestone to maintain motivation and a sense of accomplishment.

Challenge yourself: Participate in walking challenges, either on your own or with friends and family, to push yourself and add a competitive element to your walking routine.

Keep a walking journal: Record your daily step count, distance, and any thoughts or observations from your walks in a journal. Reflecting on your progress and experiences can help you stay motivated and identify any patterns or obstacles in your walking routine.

Share your progress: Share your walking achievements with friends, family, or online communities to receive support, encouragement, and accountability.

Conclusion

In conclusion, walking 10,000 steps per day is an underrated but highly effective fat-burning exercise that can complement your overall fat-loss plan. By understanding the science behind walking for fat loss, recognizing its physical and mental health benefits, and implementing strategies for increasing your daily step count, you can make walking a sustainable and enjoyable part of your journey toward achieving six-pack abs.

In the next sections of this book, we will delve into the essential components of an effective exercise routine and explore healthy recipes that can support your fat loss goals. With the combined power of walking, fasting, exercise, and a nutritious diet, you will be well-equipped to reveal your hidden six-pack abs and maintain a lean, toned physique.

Part 5: The Six-Pack Abs Workout Plan

In this chapter, we will outline a comprehensive six-pack abs workout plan designed to help you achieve the toned, sculpted abs you've always wanted. By following this plan, you'll be well on your way to revealing your hidden six-pack and creating a balanced, strong, and healthy physique. The plan focuses on the importance of a well-rounded exercise routine, incorporating warm-up and cool-down routines, targeted core exercises, cardio workouts, and strength training.

Importance of a Well-Rounded Exercise Routine

A well-rounded exercise routine is essential for achieving six-pack abs, as it ensures that you're not only working your abdominal muscles but also maintaining overall strength and conditioning. This balance is crucial for preventing injuries, promoting functional fitness, and enhancing your physical appearance. A comprehensive workout plan should include:

Warm-up and cool-down routines: These are necessary to prepare your body for exercise and prevent injuries.

Core exercises: Targeted movements that focus on strengthening and sculpting your abdominal muscles.

Cardio workouts: Activities that improve cardiovascular endurance, burn calories, and support fat loss.